Paleo
77 Delicious Paleo Recipes with an Easy Guide for Rapid Weight Loss

Introduction

I want to thank you and commend you for opening the book, "Low Carb: 77 Delicious Low Carb Recipes with an Easy Guide for Rapid Weight Loss".

This book contains proven steps and strategies to help you discover the virtues of the Paleo lifestyle. Here, you will have an increase realization about the benefits of healthy eating and keeping at it for good. Food can provide much more than daily nourishment. It can be more than that! Whatever you eat and put into your body has the power to prevent and cure illnesses, from stroke, heart diseases, and even diabetes. Therefore, it is your primary responsibility to take charge of the food you put into your mouth and in your body. This is equally the same as with the dishes you serve to your family.

In this book you will learn different kinds of Paleo recipes to help you eat smarter and get the most out of food. When we say eat smarter, it simply means eating Paleo. The basic principle behind this dietary framework is to follow our hunter-gatherer ancestors, and that is to eat food in its natural state because they simply fit humans genetically—to eat fresh, naturally-raised animals, and wild caught fish and seafood.

Let this guide be your first step towards your journey towards your 7-Day Paleo Plan, and onwards. And because you surely do not want to eat something that is not pleasing to the palate, the recipes you will find here are all enjoyable and are equally delicious. Now is the time to take charge of your health and well-being, a perfect time to change your lifestyle, the Paleo way. You sure will not regret this decision.

Thanks again for opening this book, I hope you enjoy it!

Table of Contents

Chapter 1 - Paleo Starters and Soups

1. Spicy Cashews

Ingredients:
- 2 cups whole raw cashews
- ½ teaspoon cayenne pepper
- ½ teaspoon chili powder
- ¼ teaspoon ground cinnamon
- 1 teaspoon extra-virgin olive oil
- Pinch of sea salt

Directions:

1. Mix cashew nuts, cayenne pepper, chili powder, and cinnamon in a slow cooker stoneware. Stir well. Cover and cook on high for 1 ½ hours or until nuts are toasted.

2. Meanwhile, in a bowl, combine olive oil and salt. Add to the nuts in the slow cooker and stir well to combine. Transfer to a serving bowl. Serve.

2. Sweet Orange Pecans

Ingredients:
- 1 tablespoon orange zest, grated

- ¼ cup maple syrup

- Pinch of cayenne pepper

- ½ teaspoon ground cinnamon

- 2 cups raw pecans, halved

- Pinch of sweet paprika

Directions:
1. Combine orange zest, maple syrup, cayenne pepper, and ground cinnamon in a slow cooker stoneware. Cover and cook on high for 30 minutes.

2. Stir in the pecans. Place clean towel on top of the stoneware to help absorb the moisture. Cover and cook on high for 1 hour, or until toasted.

3. Spread pecans on a baking sheet. Sprinkle with paprika and allow to cool. Serve.

3. Roasted Almonds with Thyme

Ingredients:
- 2 cups whole raw almonds, unblanched

- 1.2 teaspoon white pepper

- 2 tablespoons olive oil

- 2 tablespoons thyme

- Pinch of sea salt

Directions:
1. Combine almonds and white pepper in a slow cooker stoneware. Cover the lid and cook on high for 2 ½ hours.

2. Meanwhile, in a bowl, mix together olive oil, thyme, and salt. Add to the almonds in the slow cooker. Stir thoroughly until well combined. Spoon into a small bowl. Serve.

4. Garlic Anchovy Dip

Ingredients:
- ¾ cup extra-virgin olive oil

- 2 cloves garlic, minced

- 6 anchovy fillets, finely chopped

- Pinch of pepper

Directions:
1. Combine olive oil, garlic, anchovy fillets, and pepper in a pan. Cook for 30 minutes or until anchovies have begun to dissolve. Stir well.

2. Arrange crudités on a serving plate and serve with this dip.

5. Roasted Garlic

Ingredients:
- 2 tablespoons extra-virgin olive oil

- 20 cloves garlic, peeled

Directions:
1. Lay parchment paper and mound garlic in the middle. Spoon the olive oil all over the garlic.

2. Fold parchment paper to form a seal. Continue folding until flush with garlic. For the remaining sides to form package.

3. Put in the stoneware seam side down. Cover and cook on high for 4 hours or until caramelized.

6. Curry Parsnip Soup

Ingredients:
- 1 tablespoon extra-virgin olive oil
- 4 cloves garlic, minced
- 2 onions, finely chopped
- 2 teaspoons ground cumin
- 1 teaspoon ground coriander
- Pinch of sea salt
- Pinch of pepper
- 1 bay leaf
- 1 cinnamon stick
- 6 cups vegetable stock
- 4 cups parsnips, peeled
- ½ cup coconut milk
- 2 teaspoons curry powder
- 2 cups sweet green peas

Directions:
1. In a pan set over medium heat, pour the oil. Swirl to coat. Sauté the garlic and onions until tender and translucent. Add cumin, coriander, salt, pepper, bay leaf, and cinnamon stick. Stir

for 2 minutes. Transfer to the slow cooker. Add stock.

2. Stir in the parsnip. Cover and cook on low for 6 hours or on high for 3 hours. Discard bay leaf and cinnamon stick. Puree soup in the blender, in batches.

3. Add coconut milk. Curry powder, and green peas. Cover and cook on high for another 15 minutes. Ladle into soup bowls. Serve.

7. Fennel and Celery Soup

Ingredients:
- 2 tablespoons extra-virgin olive oil
- 2 onions, finely chopped
- 1 bulb fennel, chopped
- 4 cups celery, diced
- 1 teaspoon thyme
- 3 cloves garlic, minced
- Pinch of sea salt
- Pinch of pepper
- 5 cups vegetable stock
- ½ cup chives, finely chopped

Directions:
1. Pour oil in the pan. Swirl to coat. Sauté onions, fennel, and celery for 5 minutes or until softened. Add thyme, garlic, salt and pepper. Sauté for 2 minutes. Season with salt and pepper.

2. Pour the stock. Bring to a boil. Remove pan from heat. Puree soup using an immersion blender.

3. Ladle into soup bowls. Garnish with chives.

8. Cabbage Soup

Ingredients:
- 1 tablespoon extra-virgin olive oil
- 2 onions, finely chopped
- 2 carrots, diced
- 3 stalks celery, diced
- 3 garlic cloves, minced
- 1 teaspoon caraway seeds
- Pinch of sea salt
- Pinch of peppercorns
- 1 can tomatoes with juice
- 3 beets, diced
- 1 tablespoon coconut sugar
- 4 cups beef stock
- 3 cups cabbage, shredded
- 1 tablespoon apple cider vinegar
- ½ cup dill, finely chopped

Directions:
1. Put oil in a pan set over medium heat. Swirl to coat. Sauté onions, carrots, and celery for 5 minutes. Stir in garlic and caraway seeds. Season with salt and pepper.

2. Transfer to a blender and process until smooth. Put the soup back into the pan and add tomatoes, beets, and coconut sugar. Add the stock.

3. Cover and cook for 1 hour. Add cabbage and vinegar. Stir continuously.

4. Ladle into soup bowls and garnish with dill. Serve.

9. Mushroom Soup

Ingredients:
- 1 cup hot water
- 1 package porcini mushrooms, dried
- 1 tablespoon extra-virgin olive oil
- 2 carrots, diced
- 2 stalks celery, diced
- 2 leeks, diced
- 2 gloves garlic, minced
- Pinch of sea salt
- Pinch of peppercorns
- 1 bay leaf
- 1 cup shitake mushrooms, thinly sliced
- 1 cup cremini mushrooms, quartered
- 1 cup water
- 5 cups mushroom stock
- ½ cup chives, chopped

Directions:
1. Add hot water and mushrooms in a bowl. Let stand for 30 minutes. Drain using a fine sieve. Pat mushrooms dry using a paper towel. Chop finely. Set aside.

2. In a pan set over medium heat, pour olive oil. Swirl to coat. Add carrots, celery, and leeks. Cook for 5 minutes or until tender. Stir in garlic, salt, pepper, and bay leaf. Add mushrooms and stir for 2 minutes.

3. Pour the stock. Cook for 1 hour. Reduce heat and allow to simmer for 10 minutes. Discard bay leaf.

4. Ladle into individual soup bowls. Garnish with chives. Serve.

10. Celery Root and Watercress Soup

Ingredients:
- 2 tablespoons extra-virgin olive oil

- 3 leeks, coarsely chopped

- 2 cloves garlic, minced

- Pinch of sea salt

- Pinch of peppercorns

- 5 cups vegetable stock

- 1 celery root, sliced

- 2 bunches watercress, stems removed

- ½ cup toasted walnuts, chopped

Directions:
1. Heat oil in a pan. Sauté leeks for 5 minutes or until softened. Add the garlic, salt and pepper. Pour the stock.

2. Add the celery root. Stir well. Cover and cook for 1 hour. Add watercress, in batches.

3. Put the soup in a blender and puree until smooth. Transfer to a soup bowl. Season with salt and pepper. Refrigerate for 1 hour, or until chilled.

4. Ladle into soup bowls. Garnish with walnuts.

11. Chicken Gumbo with Okra

Ingredients:

- 1 tablespoon extra-virgin olive oil

- 2 onions, finely chopped

- 2 cups fresh chorizo sausage

- 3 stalks celery, diced

- 4 cloves garlic, minced

- 1 teaspoon Cajun seasoning

- Pinch of sea salt

- pinch of peppercorns

- 1 bay leaf

- 2 tablespoons tomato paste

- 1 can tomatoes with juice

- 1 lb. skinless, boneless chicken thighs

- 3 cups chicken stock

- ¼ teaspoon cayenne pepper

- 1 red bell pepper, diced

- 2 cups okra, diced

- ½ cup spring onions, diced

Directions:

1. Heat the oil in a pan over medium heat. Add onions, sausage, and leeks. Cook for 5 minutes or until sausage is cooked through. Stir in garlic, Cajun seasoning, salt, pepper, and bay leaf. Cook for 2 minutes.

2. Add the tomatoes paste and tomatoes with juice. Stir well. Pour in stock and chickens. Cover and cook for 1 hour. Add cayenne, bell pepper, and okra. Discard bay leaf. Allow to simmer for 15 minutes.

3. Ladle into soup bowls and garnish with spring onions.

12. Mexican-Style Chicken Soup

Ingredients:
- 2 onions, chopped
- 2 half chicken breast, cut in half
- 3 cups water
- 2 cups chicken stock
- 2 carrots, chopped
- 2 sprigs cilantro
- 2 stalks celery, chopped
- Pinch of sea salt
- Pinch of peppercorns
- 1 tablespoon ground cumin
- ½ cup sour cream
- 1 small avocado, sliced
- 1 lime juice, freshly squeezed
- ½ cup jalapeño, minced
- ½ cup cilantro leaves, chopped

Directions:
1. Combine onions, chicken breast, water, chicken stock, carrots, cilantro, celery, salt, and pepper in a slow cooker.

2. Cover the lid and cook on high for 3 hours. Lift chicken out and discard the skin and bones. Shred the meat. Set aside.

3. Strain the stock using a fine sieve. Discard the solids.

4. Meanwhile, in another bowl, whisk cumin and sour cream. Mix until well combined.

5. Ladle soup into bowls. Layer the shredded chicken and avocado strips. Sprinkle lemon juice. Top with a dollop of crema and garnish with jalapeño and cilantro.

13. Tuna Soup with Okra

Ingredients:
- 1 tablespoon extra-virgin olive oil
- 2 onions, finely chopped
- 3 stalks celery, diced
- 4 cloves garlic, minced
- 1 teaspoon Cajun seasoning
- Pinch of sea salt
- pinch of peppercorns
- 1 bay leaf
- 2 tablespoons tomato paste
- 1 can tomatoes with juice
- 1 lb. tuna, diced
- 3 cups chicken stock
- ¼ teaspoon cayenne pepper
- 1 red bell pepper, diced
- 2 cups okra, diced
- ½ cup spring onions, diced

Directions:
1. Heat the oil in a pan over medium heat. Add onions, sausage, and leeks. Cook for 5 minutes

or until sausage is cooked through. Stir in garlic, Cajun seasoning, salt, pepper, and bay leaf. Cook for 2 minutes.

2. Add the tomatoes paste and tomatoes with juice. Stir well. Pour in stock and tuna. Cover and cook for 1 hour. Add cayenne, bell pepper, and okra. Discard bay leaf. Allow to simmer for 15 minutes.

3. Ladle into soup bowls and garnish with spring onions.

14. Easy Chicken Soup

Ingredients:
- 2 onions, chopped

- 2 half chicken breast, cut in half

- 3 cups water

- 2 cups chicken stock

- 2 sprigs cilantro

- 2 stalks celery, chopped

- Pinch of sea salt

- Pinch of peppercorns

- 1 small avocado, sliced

- 1 lime juice, freshly squeezed

- ½ cup spring onions, chopped

Directions:
1. Combine onions, chicken breast, water, chicken stock, cilantro, celery, salt, and pepper in a slow cooker.

2. Cover with the lid and cook on high for 3 hours. Lift chicken out and discard the skin and bones. Shred the meat. Set aside.

3. Strain the stock using a fine sieve. Discard the solids.

4. Ladle soup into bowls. Layer the shredded chicken and avocado strips. Sprinkle lemon juice. Garnish with spring onions.

15. Hearty Beef Stock

Ingredients:
- 3 onions, quartered
- 3 stalks celery
- 3 carrots, cut into chunks
- 2 tablespoons extra-virgin olive oil
- 3 lbs. beef bones
- 12 cups water
- 1 tablespoon apple cider vinegar
- 3 sprigs thyme
- 3 sprigs parsley
- 10 black peppercorns

Directions:
1. In a roasting pan, put onions, celery, and carrots. Pour olive oil. Add the bones and toss well. Layer the ingredients in a roasting pan and roast for 1 hour.

2. Transfer to the slow cooker. Pour water, vinegar, thyme, parsley, and black peppercorns. Cook on high for 6 hours. Strain through fine sieve and discard solids.

3. Let cool and then refrigerate for 5 days or freeze in portions in airtight containers.

16. Yummy Chicken Stock

Ingredients:
- 3 onions, quartered
- 3 stalks celery
- 3 carrots, cut into chunks
- 2 tablespoons extra-virgin olive oil
- 3 lbs. bone-in skin-on chicken parts
- 12 cups water
- 1 tablespoon apple cider vinegar
- 3 sprigs thyme
- 3 sprigs parsley
- 10 black peppercorns

Directions:
1. In a roasting pan, put onions, celery, and carrots. Pour olive oil. Add the chicken parts and toss well. Layer the ingredients in a roasting pan and roast for 1 hour.

2. Transfer to the slow cooker. Pour water, vinegar, thyme, parsley, and black peppercorns. Cook on high for 6 hours. Strain through a fine sieve and discard solids.

3. Let cool and then refrigerate for 5 days or freeze in portions in airtight containers.

17. Homemade Vegetable Stock

Ingredients:
- 3 onions, quartered

- 3 stalks celery

- 3 carrots, cut into chunks

- 2 garlic cloves

- 2 bay leaves

- 12 cups water

- 1 tablespoon apple cider vinegar

- 3 sprigs thyme

- 3 sprigs parsley

- 10 black peppercorns

Directions:
1. Preheat the oven to 425 F. In a baking sheet, layer the onions, celery, and carrots. Pour olive oil. Add the garlic cloves and bay leaf. Roast for 20 minutes.

2. Transfer to the slow cooker. Pour water, vinegar, thyme, parsley, and black peppercorns. Cook on high for 6 hours. Strain through fine sieve and discard solids.

3. Let cool, and then refrigerate for 5 days or freeze portions in airtight containers.

18. Fish Stock

Ingredients:
- 12 cups water
- 3 lbs. fish trimmings, including heads
- 1 tablespoon apple cider vinegar
- 3 onions, quartered
- 3 stalks celery
- 3 carrots, cut into chunks
- 3 sprigs thyme
- 2 bay leaves
- 2 teaspoon fennel seeds
- 3 sprigs parsley
- 10 black peppercorns

Directions:
1. In a slow cooker, pour water, fish trimmings, vinegar, onions, celery, carrots, thyme, bay leaves, fennel seeds, parsley, and peppercorns.

2. Cover the lid and cook on low for 8 hours or on high for 4 hours. Discard solids and strain through fine sieve.

3. Let cool and then refrigerate for 5 days or freeze in portions in airtight containers.

19. Mushroom Stock

Ingredients:
- 12 cups water
- 1 package dried Portobello mushrooms, crumbled
- 3 onions, quartered
- 3 garlic cloves, chopped
- 3 stalks celery
- 3 carrots, cut into chunks
- 2 bay leaves
- 3 sprigs parsley
- 10 black peppercorns

Directions:
1. In a bowl, combine hot water and mushrooms. Let stand for 30 minutes.

2. Meanwhile, sauté onions, garlic, and celery. Cook for 5 minutes or until tender. Add the celery, carrots, bay leaves, parsley, and peppercorns. Cook for 3 minutes. Add the mushrooms and sauté for 1 minute.

3. Transfer to a slow cooker. Cover the lid and cook on high for 4 hours. Discard solids and strain through fine sieve.

4. Let cool and then refrigerate for 5 days or freeze in portions in airtight containers.

20. Cranberry Soup

Ingredients:
- 4 garlic cloves, chopped

- 5 cups vegetable stock

- 5 beets, coarsely chopped, set aside leaves

- Pinch of sea salt

- Pinch of peppercorns

- 2 tablespoons coconut sugar

- 1 cup cranberries

- 1 orange juice, freshly squeezed

- 1 orange zest

- ½ cup fresh dill fronds, chopped

Directions:
1. In a large saucepan, combine garlic, stock, beets, salt, and pepper. Cover the lid and cook on low for 6 hours.

2. Stir in coconut sugar, cranberries, orange juice and zest, and beet leaves. Cover again and cook on high for 30 minutes.

3. Puree the soup in a blender. Transfer to a large soup bow and chill overnight

4. When ready to sue, ladle into individual bowls. Garnish with dill.

Chapter 2 – Paleo Fish and Seafood

21. Braised Swordfish with Black Olives

Ingredients:
- 2 large swordfish steaks

- 1 sweet onion, thinly sliced

- 2 cloves garlic, minced

- 1 teaspoon chili powder

- ½ cup parsley leaves, chopped

- Pinch of sea salt

- Pinch of pepper

- ½ cup extra-virgin olive oil

- 1 ½ cups apple cider vinegar

Directions:
1. In a pan, put the swordfish. Sprinkle with onion, garlic, chili powder, parsley, salt, and pepper. Pour olive oil until the fish is coated. Pour apple cider vinegar. Cook for 1 hour or until the fish is flaky.

2. Lift out fish and cut in half. Serve.

22. Poached Halibut

Ingredients:
Poaching Liquid
- 6 cups water

- ½ cup lemon juice

- 1 onion, chopped

- 2 bay leaves

- 2 stalks celery, chopped, leaves included

- 2 sprigs parsley

- Pinch of sea salt

- Pinch of pepper

For the halibut
- 2 lbs. halibut fillets

Directions:
1. For the poaching liquid, combine water, lemon juice, onion, bay leaves, celery, parsley, salt, and pepper. Bring to a boil and allow to simmer for 20 minutes. Strain and discard solids.

2. For the halibut, add the poaching liquid in a pan. Put the halibut fillets. Cook for 45 minutes or until the fish is flaky. Transfer to a soup bowl. Discard bay leaves. Serve.

23. Braised Red Snapper

Ingredients:
- 2 large red snapper steaks

- 1 sweet onion, thinly sliced

- 2 cloves garlic, minced

- 1 teaspoon chili powder

- ½ cup parsley leaves, chopped

- Pinch of sea salt

- Pinch of pepper

- ½ cup extra-virgin olive oil

- 1 ½ cups apple cider vinegar

Directions:
1. In a pan, put the red snapper. Sprinkle with onion, garlic, chili powder, parsley, salt, and pepper. Pour olive oil until the fish is coated. Pour apple cider vinegar. Cook for 1 hour or until the fish is flaky.

2. Lift out fish and cut in half. Serve.

24. Poached Salmon

Ingredients:
Poaching Liquid
- 6 cups water

- ½ cup lemon juice

- 1 onion, chopped

- 2 bay leaves

- 2 stalks celery, chopped, leaves included

- 2 sprigs parsley

- Pinch of sea salt

- Pinch of pepper

For the salmon
- 2 lbs. salmon fillets

Directions:
1. For the poaching liquid, combine water, lemon juice, onion, bay leaves, celery, parsley, salt, and pepper. Bring to a boil and allow to simmer for 20 minutes. Strain and discard solids.

2. For the salmon, add the poaching liquid in a pan. Put the salmon fillets. Cook for 45 minutes or until the fish is flaky. Transfer to a soup bowl. Discard bay leaves. Serve.

25. Creamy and Spicy Coconut Grouper

Ingredients:
- 2 lbs. skinless grouper fillets

- 1 cup cilantro leaves, chopped

- ¼ teaspoon cayenne pepper

- 2 tablespoons lime juice, freshly squeezed

- 2 tablespoons olive oil

- 2 onions, finely chopped

- 3 cloves garlic, minced

- 2 stalks celery, diced

- 1 teaspoon dried oregano

- Pinch of sea salt

- Pinch of peppercorns

- 1 can tomatoes with juice, diced

- 1 cup fish stock

- 1 can coconut milk

- 2 red chili peppers, minced

Directions:
1. Combine grouper fillets, cilantro, cayenne, and lime juice in a bowl. Mix well.

2. Meanwhile, heat the oil in a pan. Swirl to coat. Sauté onions and garlic for 3 minutes. Stir in celery and oregano. Season with salt and pepper. Cook for 2 minutes. Pour tomatoes with juice. Bring to a boil.

3. Add grouper fillets, fish stock, coconut milk, and chili peppers. Cook for 45 minutes or until the fish is flaky and the mixture hot and bubbly. Serve.

26. Poached Tuna

Ingredients:
Poaching Liquid
- 6 cups water

- ½ cup lemon juice

- 1 onion, chopped

- 2 bay leaves

- 2 stalks celery, chopped, leaves included

- 2 sprigs parsley

- Pinch of sea salt

- Pinch of pepper

For the tuna
- 2 lbs. tuna fillets

Directions:
3. For the poaching liquid, combine water, lemon juice, onion, bay leaves, celery, parsley, salt, and pepper. Bring to a boil and allow to simmer for 20 minutes. Strain and discard solids.

4. For the tuna, add the poaching liquid in a pan. Put the tuna fillets. Cook for 45 minutes or until the fish is flaky. Transfer to a soup bowl. Discard bay leaves. Serve.

27. Spiced Coconut Tuna in Coconut Milk

Ingredients:
- 2 lbs. tuna fillets
- 1 cup cilantro leaves, chopped
- ¼ teaspoon cayenne pepper
- 2 tablespoons lime juice, freshly squeezed
- 2 tablespoons olive oil
- 2 onions, finely chopped
- 3 cloves garlic, minced
- 2 stalks celery, diced
- 1 teaspoon dried oregano
- Pinch of sea salt
- Pinch of peppercorns
- 1 can tomatoes with juice, diced
- 1 cup fish stock
- 1 can coconut milk
- 2 red chili peppers, minced

Directions:
1. Combine tuna fillets, cilantro, cayenne, and lime juice in a bowl. Mix well.

2. Meanwhile, heat the oil in a pan. Swirl to coat. Sauté onions and garlic for 3 minutes. Stir in celery and oregano. Season with salt and pepper. Cook for 2 minutes. Pour tomatoes with juice. Bring to a boil.

3. Add tuna fillets, fish stock, coconut milk, and chili peppers. Cook for 45 minutes or until the fish is flaky and the mixture hot and bubbly. Serve.

28. Spiced Salmon with Spinach

Ingredients:
- 2 tablespoons lemon juice, freshly squeezed
- ¼ teaspoon cayenne pepper
- 1 teaspoon garam marsala
- 1 ½ lbs. salmon fillets
- 3 garlic cloves, minced
- 2 onions, finely chopped
- 1 tablespoon gingerroot, minced
- ½ teaspoon turmeric
- 1 tablespoon ground cumin
- 1 tablespoon ground coriander
- Pinch of sea salt
- Pinch of peppercorns
- 1 can tomatoes with juice
- 3 cups spinach leaves

Directions:
1. Mix together lemon juice, cayenne, and garam masala in a bowl. Add the salmon fillets and toss well to combine.

2. In a pan set over medium heat, pour the oil. Swirl to coat. Add the garlic, onions, gingerroot, turmeric, cumin, coriander, salt, and pepper. Stir for 3 minutes. Add the tomatoes with juice. Bring to a boil.

3. Stir in the spinach. Allow to simmer for 15 minutes. Add the reserved salmon juices and cook for 30 minutes or until the fish is flaky. Serve.

29. Fish Stew with Anchovies

Ingredients:
- 1 tablespoon extra-virgin olive oil

- 2 onions, finely chopped

- 1 bulb fennel, diced

- 3 cloves garlic, minced

- 2 teaspoons dried Italian seasoning

- 1 teaspoon sea salt

- 1 teaspoon peppercorns

- 1 can diced tomatoes with juice

- 2 cups fish stock

- ½ cup black olives, chopped

- 1 ½ lbs. firm white fish, such as halibut

- 1 jalapeño pepper, diced

Directions:
1. Heat the oil in a pan set over medium high. Swirl to coat. Sauté the onions and fennel for 3 minutes. Add the garlic, Italian seasoning, salt, and pepper. Sauté for 2 minutes. Add tomatoes with juice and bring to a boil.

2. Transfer to a slow cooker. Pour the fish stock. Cover the lid and cook on low for 6 hours or on

high for 3 hours. Add the olives, fish, and jalapeno pepper. Cover the lid and cook on high for 10 minutes.

3. Ladle stew into soup bowls. Serve.

30. Haddock with Spinach

Ingredients:
- 2 tablespoons lemon juice, freshly squeezed
- ¼ teaspoon cayenne pepper
- 1 teaspoon garam marsala
- 2 lbs. haddock steak
- 3 garlic cloves, minced
- 2 onions, finely chopped
- 1 tablespoon gingerroot, minced
- ½ teaspoon turmeric
- 1 tablespoon ground cumin
- 1 tablespoon ground coriander
- Pinch of sea salt
- Pinch of peppercorns
- 1 can tomatoes with juice
- 3 cups spinach leaves

Directions:
1. Mix together lemon juice, cayenne, and garam masala in a bowl. Add the haddock steaks and toss well to combine.

2. In a pan set over medium heat, pour the oil. Swirl to coat. Add the garlic, onions, gingerroot, turmeric, cumin, coriander, salt, and pepper. Stir for 3 minutes. Add the tomatoes with juice. Bring to a boil.

3. Stir in the spinach. Allow to simmer for 15 minutes. Add the reserved haddock juices and cook for 30 minutes or until the fish is flaky. Serve.

31. Coconut Shrimp Curry

Ingredients:
- 1 lb. shrimp, deveined

- 2 tablespoons lemon juice, freshly squeezed

- ½ teaspoon turmeric

- 1 teaspoon ground cumin

- 2 teaspoons ground coriander

- ½ teaspoon sea salt

- ¼ teaspoon cayenne pepper

Chapter 3 – Paleo Vegetable Dinners

32. Sweet and Sour Sprouts

Ingredients:
- 1 lb. frozen baby sprouts

- 2 cups stock

- ½ cup apple cider vinegar

- 1 ½ tablespoons tomato ketchup

- 1 tablespoon teriyaki sauce

- 1 ½ tablespoons hoisin sauce

- 1 tablespoon corn flour

Directions:
1. In a pan, put the sprouts together with the stock. Stir occasionally. Let it simmer or until the sprouts are cooked just the way you liked them. Drain and set aside. Pour stock in the pan.

2. Add apple cider vinegar, ketchup, teriyaki sauce, and hoisin sauce. Bring to a boil. When boiling, add the corn flour and water paste. Let it boil and thicken.

3. Stir in the sprouts. Serve warm.

33. Stir-Fried Broccoli

Ingredients:
- 1 lb. broccoli stalks

- 3 black olives

- Pinch dried chilies

- 2 garlic cloves, crushed

- ½ teaspoon ground coriander

- ½ teaspoon ground cumin

- 2 sun-dried tomatoes

- ½ tablespoons capers

- Juice of 1 lemon

- ½ silver rind lemon

- 3 cups stock

- ½ teaspoon olive brine

- ½ teaspoon caper brine

- Pinch of salt

- Pinch of pepper

Directions:
1. Slice the stalks into thin rounds. Make sure to cut the woody bottoms.

2. In a pan, combine olives, chilies, garlic, coriander, cumin, sun-dried tomatoes, capers, lemon juice, lemon rind, half the stock, olive and caper brines. Bring into a boil and reduce heat.

3. Wait until the liquid is syrupy before adding the broccoli stalks. Pour the remaining stock and ½ lemon juice. Stir fry until the broccoli is tender. Season with salt and pepper. Serve.

34. Spicy Cauliflower in Tomato Sauce

Ingredients:
- 2 cloves garlic, crushed
- 2 black olives, drained
- ½ teaspoon rosemary
- 2 generous pinches of dried chilies
- 1 teaspoon fennel seeds
- 3 cups stock
- 1 red bell pepper
- 1 yellow bell pepper
- 2 tablespoons tomato puree
- Pinch of salt
- Pinch of pepper
- 2 tablespoons parsley, chopped

Directions:
1. In a pan, combine garlic, olives, rosemary, dried chilies, fennel seeds, half the stock, bell peppers. Bring to a boil. Reduce the heat to low and let it simmer for 10 minutes.

2. Add the cauliflower, tomato puree, and the remaining stock. Put salt and pepper and let it

simmer for 15 minutes. Stir until the cauliflower is tender. Serve with parsley on top.

35. Pan-Braised Fennel

Ingredients:
- 2 bulbs fennel

- 2 cups stock

- Pinch of salt

- Pinch of pepper

Directions:
1. Trim the tough layers, leaves and stalks from the bulbs. Save the fronds to use as garnish, and the trimmings to make the stock. Just make sure to keep the core intact.

2. Cut the fennel bulbs into halves. Place cut-side downs in a pan. Pour the stock. Season with salt and pepper. Let it simmer until glazed. If the fennel cooked a bit faster, remove and set aside. If the liquid cooks away, add more stocks or water. Serve.

36. Grilled Courgettes

Ingredients:
- 5 courgettes, sliced in ¼ inch
- Olive oil spray

Directions:
1. Preheat the grill to high heat. Mist a non-stick baking sheet with olive oil.

2. Spread the slices of courgette on the baking sheet. Mist the slices with the oil and grill for 5 minutes. Do the same thing on the other side.

37. Chinese Style Cauliflower

Ingredients:
- 2 garlic cloves, crushed
- 5 spring onions, thinly sliced
- 1 root ginger, thinly sliced
- 4 cups stock
- 2 tablespoons dry sherry
- ½ juice of orange
- 12 cauliflower florets, steamed
- 2 tablespoons hoisin sauce
- 1 tablespoon coriander, chopped

Directions:
1. In a pan, combine the garlic, onions, ginger, stock, and sherry. Let it simmer until the garlic and onions are tender, and the liquid is almost gone.

2. Pour the orange juice and stir in the cauliflower. Cook for 3 minutes and then add the hoisin sauce. Cook until well combined. Sprinkle with coriander before serving.

38. Corn and Mushroom

Ingredients:
- 3 spring onions, sliced

- 4 button mushrooms sliced

- 3 cups stock

- 2 dashes teriyaki sauce

- 1 tablespoon dry sherry

- 200 grams can sweetcorn kernels, drained

- 1 tablespoon fresh parsley, chopped

Directions:
1. In a small pan, combine the onions, mushrooms, stock, teriyaki sauce, and sherry. Let it simmer until the mushrooms are tender.

2. Spread the corn and parsley and cook for 2 minutes. Serve.

39. Mushrooms in Teriyaki Sauce

Ingredients:
- 1 lb. mushrooms

- 3 cups stock

- 3 cups sherry

- 2 tablespoons teriyaki sauce

- Pinch of salt

- Pinch of pepper

Directions:
1. In a pan, put the mushrooms and sauté. Immediately stir the sherry and sashes of teriyaki. Simmer briskly or until the mushrooms have release liquid.

2. Reduce heat and let it simmer until the liquid has been absorbed. Season with salt and pepper. Serve.

40. Sweet and Sour Onions

Ingredients:
- 5 large onions, halved

- 2 garlic cloves, crushed

- ½ teaspoon Dijon mustard

- 3 cups stock

- 1 tablespoon sugar

- 1 ½ tablespoon balsamic vinegar

Directions:
1. In a pan, put the onions and garlic. Sauté until both are tender. Add the mustard, stock, sugar, and vinegar. Bring to a boil.

2. Reduce heat. Cover and let it simmer for 10 minutes.

3. Remove from heat. Continue stirring until the onions are brown and the liquid is reduced. Serve.

41. Sautéed Onions and Apples

Ingredients:
- 1 large onion, halved

- 2 cups dry cider

- 4 tart eating apples, sliced into wedges

- 2 cups stock

- Pinch pf salt

- Pinch of pepper

Directions:
1. In a saucepan, combine the onion and cider. Let it boil or until the onions are cooked and liquid almost gone.

2. Stir in the apples and stock. Season with salt and pepper. Stir occasionally. Scrape brown bits from the bottom of the pan. Cook for 10 minutes or until the apples are tender and not mushy.

42. Mixed Veggies in Garlic Oil

Ingredients:
- 2 onions, unpeeled
- 2 red bell peppers
- 2 green bell peppers
- 2 large tomatoes
- 3 cloves garlic, peeled
- ¼ cup extra-virgin olive oil
- 1 eggplant
- 1 zucchini
- Pinch of salt
- Pinch of pepper
- 2 tablespoons basil
- ¼ cup red wine vinegar

Directions:
1. Preheat the grill to medium high.

2. Put the red onions, unpeeled outside of the grate. Make sure they are over indirect heat. Cook until slightly charred. Remove. Once cooled, discard charred layers. Place peppers and tomatoes over the flames and cook until slightly charred.

3. Meanwhile, in a saucepan, combine olive oil and garlic. Cook until the garlic is golden brown.

4. Rub the eggplant and zucchini with olive oil. Season with salt and pepper. Grill until cooked through.

5. When all vegetables have been grilled, cut them in uniform slices. Place in a platter and drizzle with garlic oil, basil, and red wine vinegar. Mix and serve.

43. Sautéed Green Tomato

Ingredients:
- ¼ cup coconut flour

- Pinch of salt

- Pinch of pepper

- 4 green tomatoes2 eggs

- ½ cup parmesan cheese

- ½ cup almond flour

- ¼ cup olive oil

Directions:
1. In a bowl, combine the coconut flour, salt, and pepper. Mix the tomatoes. Toss until coated.

2. Beat the eggs in another bowl. Add the almond flour and parmesan cheese. Combine well.

3. Heat the oil. Dip the tomatoes into the egg mixture and into the parmesan and almond mixture. Fry them in batches until golden brown. Serve.

44. Mixed Vegetables

Ingredients:
- 3 tablespoons vegetable oil

- 1 package of mixed frozen vegetables such as red bell peppers, green beans, broccoli, and mushrooms

- 2 tablespoons soy sauce

- 2 tablespoons water

- 1 package fresh spinach

Directions:
1. In a pan, heat 1 ½ tablespoons olive oil. Pour frozen vegetables and sauté for 5 minutes or until all vegetables are tender. Add soy sauce and water and cook for another 3 minutes. Add the spinach.

2. Let the veggies cook over medium heat for 3 minutes. Turn the spinach once so it heats evenly. Cover and steam for an additional 2 minutes.

3. Ladle into a bowl and pour the vegetables. Serve.

45. Baked Tomatoes in Tofutti Cheese

Ingredients:
- 3 large tomatoes, cut in half

- ¼ cup fresh herbs (parsley, basil and marjoram)

- ½ cup Tofutti cheese

- ½ cup grated bread crumbs

- 2 cloves garlic, minced

- Pinch of salt

- Pinch of pepper

- 3 tablespoons extra-virgin olive oil

Directions:
1. Preheat the oven to 350 F. Put the tomatoes in a baking dish.

2. Combine the herbs (parsley, basil, and marjoram), Tofutti cheese, bread crumbs, garlic, salt, pepper, and oil in a bowl. Mix well.

3. Sprinkle each tomato with an equal portion of the mixture. Bake for 30 minutes. Serve.

46. Veggie Toast

Ingredients:
- 3 zucchinis, sliced
- 2 leeks, chopped
- 2 tablespoons extra-virgin olive oil
- 2 green peppers, sliced
- Vegan pesto
- 25g vegetarian Parmesan-style cheese, grated
- 1 thick slice white bread
- 50g shelled pistachios
- 1 tablespoon olive oil

Directions:
1. Preheat the oven to 400 F.

2. Combine the zucchini, leeks, and pepper in both the pesto and oil. Bake the vegetables for 20 minutes. Stir the veggies and bake for another 20 minutes.

3. Meanwhile, in a food processor, mix the Parmesan-style cheese, bread, pistachios, and oil until it forms a rough crumb. Top the vegetables with crumbs and bake for another 15 minutes or until crisp and golden brown.

47. Vegetable Salad in Basil Vinaigrette

Ingredients:
- ½ cup basil leaves

- 1 tablespoon sugar

- Pinch of salt

- 3 tablespoons vinegar

- 1 teaspoon Dijon mustard

- 4 ears of corn

- 1 cup green beans

- 1 ½ cup cucumber, chopped

- 5 tablespoons green onions, thinly sliced

- 1 cup cherry tomatoes, halved

- ½ cup red sweet pepper

Directions:
1. For the vinaigrette, put basil, sugar, and salt in the food processor. Process until the basil is finely chopped. Add the vinegar and mustard. Process until you achieve a smooth consistency.

2. In a pan, cook the corn and green beans for 5 minutes in a boiling water. Rinse with cold water.

3. In a bowl, put the cucumber, green onions, tomatoes, and pepper. Stir in the corn and green beans. Drizzle the vinaigrette over the vegetables. Toss to coat and let sit for 15 minutes before serving.

48. Grilled Asparagus and Citrus Quarters

Ingredients:
- 1 orange

- 1 lemon

- 2 tablespoons olive oil

- Pinch of salt

- Pinch of pepper

- 2 lbs. asparagus spears

- 16 sea scallops

- 1 teaspoon lemon-pepper seasoning

Directions:
1. Cut the orange and lemon into quarters. Set aside.

2. Combine the olive oil, salt, and pepper in a bowl.

3. Cover and grill asparagus for 10 minutes or until crisp-tender. Remove and set aside.

4. In a bowl, mix the citrus peels, oil, and lemon-pepper mixture. Marinade for 10 minutes. Grill the citrus quarters for 2 minutes.

5. Combine asparagus and citrus fruits in a platter and serve.

49. Roasted Carrots with Toasted Seeds

Ingredients:
- 1 teaspoon cumin seeds
- 1 tablespoon coriander seeds
- 1 teaspoon black onion seeds
- 2 tablespoons sesame seeds
- 1 tablespoon honey
- 3 tablespoon groundnut oil
- 2 green chilies, sliced
- 3 carrots, sliced
- 2 red onions, sliced
- Pinch of salt
- Pinch of pepper
- Handful of fresh coriander

For the dressing
- Juice of ½ lemon
- 2 tablespoons groundnut oil
- Toasted sesame oil

Directions:

1. Preheat the oven to 400 F. Cook the cumin and coriander seeds. Toast for 2 minutes then crush.

2. In the same pan, toast the onion seeds and sesame seeds. Stir and mix with honey and oil. Stir in the chilies, carrots, and onions. Mix well. Season with salt and pepper.

3. Put the vegetables into the roasting pan and roast for 20 minutes. Let cool and chill.

4. To make the dressing, mix the lemon juice, groundnut oil, and sesame oil. Put salt and pepper. Pour the dressing into the carrots. Sprinkle with coriander leaves.

50. Broccoli and Pumpkin Seeds

Ingredients:
- ½ cup water

- 5 cups broccoli florets

- 1 teaspoon olive oil

- 1 tablespoon maple syrup

- 1 tablespoon vinegar

- Pinch crushed red pepper

- ¼ cup pumpkin seeds

Directions:
1. Pour water over the skillet and bring to a boil. Add broccoli florets and cook, uncovered for 4 minutes or until the water has evaporated.

2. Put some olive oil and stir broccoli for 2 minutes. Remove and set aside.

3. Drizzle maple syrup and vinegar into the broccoli. Season with salt and pepper. Sprinkle with pumpkin seeds. Serve.

Chapter 4 – Paleo Pasta

51. Courgette and Pepper Sauce Pasta

Ingredients:

- 1 red onion, chopped

- 2 medium courgettes, chopped

- ½ pint stock

- 1 red bell pepper, chopped

- 1 yellow bell pepper, chopped

- 1 green bell pepper, chopped

- 3 black olives, drained

- 3 sundried tomatoes, chopped

- 3 garlic cloves, crushed

- 14 oz. chopped tomatoes

- 4 fl oz. tomato puree

- Parmesan cheese

- 3 tablespoons parsley, chopped

Directions:
1. In a pan, combine red onion, courgettes, stock, bell peppers, olives, sundried tomatoes, garlic, and tomatoes. Cover and bring to a boil for 7 minutes. Uncover and let it simmer until the vegetables are tender.

2. Stir in the tomatoes and tomato puree. Simmer, uncovered for 10 minutes.

3. Pour a generous serving of the sauce onto the pasta. Scatter parmesan cheese and drizzle with parsley.

52. Peppery Tomato Sauce

Ingredients:
- 3 red bell peppers
- 2 plum tomatoes, chopped
- 1 teaspoon vinegar
- 1 teaspoon oregano, minced
- Pinch of salt
- Pinch of pepper
- 1 garlic clove, chopped
- ¼ teaspoon salt

Directions:
1. Preheat the grill to medium high. Place the bell peppers on the grill rack and grill for 15 minutes. When cool enough to handle, peel the peppers and remove the seeds. Set aside.
2. In a food processor, put plum tomatoes, vinegar, oregano, salt, and pepper. Puree until smooth. Pour the mixture through a sieve and press as much liquid as you can get. Set aside.
3. Mash garlic and salt until it forms a paste. Combine with the tomato mixture. Refrigerate until ready to use.
4. The sauce can be spooned over spaghetti.

53. Courgette and Pepper Sauce Pasta

Ingredients:
- 1 red onion, chopped
- 2 medium courgettes, chopped
- ½ pint stock
- 1 red bell pepper, chopped
- 1 yellow bell pepper, chopped
- 1 green bell pepper, chopped
- 3 black olives, drained
- 3 sundried tomatoes, chopped
- 3 garlic cloves, crushed
- 14 oz. chopped tomatoes
- 4 fl oz. tomato puree
- Parmesan cheese
- -3 tablespoons parsley, chopped

Directions:
1. In a pan, combine red onion, courgettes, stock, bell peppers, olives, sundried tomatoes, garlic, and tomatoes. Cover and bring to a boil for 7 minutes. Uncover and let it simmer until the vegetables are tender.

2. Stir in the tomatoes and tomato puree. Simmer, uncovered for 10 minutes.

3. Pour a generous serving of the sauce onto the pasta. Scatter parmesan cheese and drizzle with parsley.

54. Courgette Pasta

Ingredients:
- 1 red onion, chopped
- 2 medium courgettes, chopped
- ½ pint stock
- 1 red bell pepper, chopped
- 1 yellow bell pepper, chopped
- 1 green bell pepper, chopped
- 3 black olives, drained
- 3 sundried tomatoes, chopped
- 3 garlic cloves, crushed
- 14 oz. chopped tomatoes
- 4 fl oz. tomato puree
- Parmesan cheese
- 3 tablespoons parsley, chopped

Directions:
1. In a pan, combine red onion, courgettes, stock, bell peppers, olives, sundried tomatoes, garlic, and tomatoes. Cover and bring to a boil for 7 minutes. Uncover and let it simmer until the vegetables are tender.

2. Stir in the tomatoes and tomato puree. Simmer, uncovered for 10 minutes.

3. Pour a generous serving of the sauce onto the pasta. Scatter parmesan cheese and drizzle with parsley.

55. Peppery Tomato Sauce

Ingredients:
- 3 red bell peppers
- 2 plum tomatoes, chopped
- 1 teaspoon vinegar
- 1 teaspoon oregano, minced
- Pinch of salt
- Pinch of pepper
- 1 garlic clove, chopped
- ¼ teaspoon salt

Directions:
1. Preheat the grill to medium high. Place the bell peppers on the grill rack and grill for 15 minutes. When cool enough to handle, peel the peppers and remove the seeds. Set aside.
2. In a food processor, put plum tomatoes, vinegar, oregano, salt, and pepper. Puree until smooth. Pour the mixture through a sieve and press as much liquid as you can get. Set aside.
3. Mash garlic and salt until it forms a paste. Combine with the tomato mixture. Refrigerate until ready to use.
4. The sauce can be spooned over spaghetti.

56. Tomato Pasta Sauce

Ingredients:
- 3 red bell peppers

- 2 plum tomatoes, chopped

- 1 teaspoon vinegar

- 1 teaspoon oregano, minced

- Pinch of salt

- Pinch of pepper

- 1 garlic clove, chopped

- ¼ teaspoon salt

Directions:
1. Preheat the grill to medium high. Place the bell peppers on the grill rack and grill for 15 minutes. When cool enough to handle, peel the peppers and remove the seeds. Set aside.
2. In a food processor, put plum tomatoes, vinegar, oregano, salt, and pepper. Puree until smooth. Pour the mixture through a sieve and press as much liquid as you can get. Set aside.
3. Mash garlic and salt until it forms a paste. Combine with the tomato mixture. Refrigerate until ready to use.
4. The sauce can be spooned over spaghetti.

57. Oven-Fried Chicken Thighs

Ingredients:
- Chicken thighs, skinned

- Pinch of salt

- Pinch of pepper

- Dry breadcrumbs

- Olive oil

Directions:
1. Preheat the oven to 375 F. Rub chicken with salt and pepper. Coat with breadcrumbs.
2. Line a baking sheet and spray with oil. Bake for 40 minutes. Serve.

58. Chicken Thighs

Ingredients:
- Chicken thighs, skinned

- Pinch of salt

- Pinch of pepper

- Dry breadcrumbs

- Olive oil

Directions:
1. Preheat the oven to 375 F. Rub chicken with salt and pepper. Coat with breadcrumbs.
2. Line a baking sheet and spray with oil. Bake for 40 minutes. Serve.

59. Sautéed Green Tomato

Ingredients:
- ¼ cup coconut flour

- Pinch of salt

- Pinch of pepper

- 4 green tomatoes2 eggs

- ½ cup parmesan cheese

- ½ cup almond flour

- ¼ cup olive oil

Directions:
1. In a bowl, combine the coconut flour, salt, and pepper. Mix the tomatoes. Toss until coated.
2. Beat the eggs in another bowl. Add the almond flour and parmesan cheese. Combine well.
3. Heat the oil. Dip the tomatoes into the egg mixture and into the parmesan and almond mixture. Fry them in batches until golden brown. Serve.

60. Grilled Orange Dip

Origin: United States
This dip can be best served with slices of grilled beef, boneless chicken, or fish.
Carbohydrates: 11 grams
Ingredients:

- 1 navel orange

- 1 red onion, thinly sliced

- 1 garlic clove, chopped

- ¼ teaspoon salt

- 2 teaspoons vinegar

- 1/3 cup dried cherries

- ¼ teaspoon rosemary, chopped

- Pinch of red pepper

Directions:
1. Preheat the grill to medium high.
2. Cut the orange in half. First half into ¼ inch slices. Cut off the white pith in the other. Place the slices on the grill rack and grill for 5 minutes. Transfer to a plate and set aside.
3. Meanwhile, in a serving bowl, mash the garlic and salt until it forms into a paste.
4. Mix all both grilled and raw orange slices, onion, and garlic paste. Add the vinegar, cherries, rosemary, and red pepper. Toss well. Serve.

61. Corn, Avocado, and Tomato Mix

Origin: United States
The mixture of corn, avocado, and tomato are perfect blend to serve as side dish for fish, beef, and chicken.
Carbohydrates: 11 grams
Ingredients:

- 1 ear of corn

- ½ ripe avocado, cut into chunks

- 10 grape tomatoes

- 3 basil leaves, chopped

- 3 tablespoons onion, finely chopped

- 2 teaspoons lime juice

- 2 teaspoons olive oil

- Pinch of salt

- Pinch of pepper

Directions:
1. Slice avocados into chunks and remove kernels from the corn using a knife.
2. Place them in a serving bowl. Toss tomatoes, basil leaves, onion, lime juice, olive oil, salt, and pepper.
3. Toss to mix well. Serve at once or refrigerate overnight.

62. Roasted Brussels Sprouts

Ingredients:

- Nonstick cooking spray
- 1 lb. Brussels sprouts
- 1 tablespoon olive oil
- ½ yellow onion, finely chopped
- ½ teaspoon ground black pepper

Directions:
1. Preheat the oven to 425 F. Line a baking sheet with cooking oil and place a steamer basket in a large pot. Add 1 inch of water and bring to a boil.
2. Place the Brussels sprouts in the steamer basket and steam for 4 minutes or until barely tender.
3. Remove the Brussels from the pot and drain well. Transfer to a large bowl and toss in the olive oil, onion, and pepper to coat.
4. Spread the vegetables in a single layer and bake for 15 minutes. Do not overcook.

63. Roasted Brussels Sprouts

Ingredients:

- Nonstick cooking spray

- 1 lb. Brussels sprouts

- 1 tablespoon olive oil

- ½ yellow onion, finely chopped

- ½ teaspoon ground black pepper

Directions:
1. Preheat the oven to 425 F. Line a baking sheet with cooking oil and place a steamer basket in a large pot. Add 1 inch of water and bring to a boil.
2. Place the Brussels sprouts in the steamer basket and steam for 4 minutes or until barely tender.
3. Remove the Brussels from the pot and drain well. Transfer to a large bowl and toss in the olive oil, onion, and pepper to coat.
4. Spread the vegetables in a single layer and bake for 15 minutes. Do not overcook.

64. Roasted Cauliflower

Ingredients:
- 4 cups cauliflower florets

- 4 tablespoons olive oil

- ¼ cup bread crumbs

Directions:
1. Preheat the oven to 400 F.
2. Place the cauliflower on a large baking sheet and drizzle with olive oil and sprinkle with bread crumbs. Spread out evenly in a single layer.
3. Bake for 20 minutes or until crisp-tender. Serve hot.

65. Leafy Greens Soup

Ingredients:

- 2 tablespoons extra-virgin olive oil
- 5 leeks, white and light green part, thinly sliced
- 4 cloves garlic, sliced
- ½ teaspoon salt
- ½ teaspoon pepper
- 1 teaspoon dried tarragon
- 6 cups vegetable stock
- 4 cups Swiss chard leaves
- 1 cup parsley leaves

Directions:
1. In a large skillet, heat the oil over medium heat. Toss in the leeks and cook for 5 minutes. Add the garlic, salt, pepper, and tarragon. Stir for 1 minute. Add 2 cups of stock and bring to a boil.
2. Stir in the remaining 4 cups of vegetable stock. Add the Swiss chard and sorrel in batches. Cook on high for 15 minutes or until the greens become tender.
3. Pulp using a food processor. Spoon into individual serving bowls.

66. Spinach-Stuffed Mushrooms

Ingredients:
- ½ cup water

- 1 package spinach, chopped

- 1/8 teaspoon salt

- 8 large mushrooms

- 1 tablespoon extra-virgin olive oil

Directions
1. In a medium saucepan, add 1/2 cup of water and bring to a boil. Add the spinach and salt.
2. Meanwhile, wash the mushrooms and remove the stems, trim the ends, and chop the stems.
3. Heat the olive oil in a large skillet. Add the chopped mushrooms and sauté for 3 minutes or until golden brown. Remove from the pan.
4. Add the mushroom caps and sauté for 5 minutes. Transfer to a platter.
5. Drain the spinach and stir in the sautéed mushrooms. Spoon the spinach mixture and serve immediately.

67. Stewed Onions and Tomatoes

Ingredients:
- 1 tablespoon olive oil

- 1 small onion, chopped

- 1 clove garlic, chopped

- ½ cup green bell pepper, chopped

- ¼ cup celery, thinly sliced

- 1 tablespoon balsamic vinegar

- 3 cups tomatoes, chopped

- 1/8 teaspoon ground black pepper

Directions:
1. In a large nonstick skillet, heat the oil. Sauté the onion, garlic, bell pepper, and celery for 5 minutes or until the vegetables are tender.
2. Add the vinegar, tomatoes, and pepper. Bring to a boil. Reduce the heat and let it simmer for another 10 minutes. Serve.

68. Stir-Fry Vegetables

Ingredients:
- 3 tablespoons vegetable oil

- 1 package containing frozen vegetables such as green beans, broccoli, red bell peppers, and mushrooms

- 2 tablespoons soy sauce

- 2 tablespoons water

- 1 package fresh spinach

Directions:
1. In a large skillet, heat 1 ½ tablespoons olive oil. Add the frozen vegetables and stir fry for about 5 minutes or until all vegetables are tender. Add soy sauce and water and stir-fry for another 3 minutes. Add the spinach
2. Cover the pan and let it steam over medium heat for 3 minutes. Turn the spinach once so it heats evenly. Cover and steam for an additional 2 minutes.
3. Spoon the liquid into a bowl and pour in the vegetables. Serve.

69. Zucchini Spaghetti Squash

Ingredients:
- spaghetti squash, seeded and halved lengthwise

- 2 tablespoons olive oil

- 2 small red onion

- 1 zucchini

- ¼ teaspoon salt

- 4 tomatoes, cubed

- ¼ teaspoon ground pepper

- 1 lemon, sliced

Directions:
1. In a baking dish, place the squash halves. Add ¼ cup of water and wrap with a plastic wrap. Put the dish on the microwave and set for 10 minutes on high or until tender. Remove and let it cool.
2. Meanwhile, in a skillet, warm the oil and cook the onion. Sauté for 3 minutes or until translucent. Toss in the zucchini and cook for 5 minutes or until the color turns to brown.
3. Toss in the tomatoes, salt, and pepper. Let it simmer for 10 minutes.

4. Transfer the squash strands into a dish and put the remaining oil. In a pasta bowl, pile the squash in the center and put a dollop of veggie mix around the squash. Add the slices of lemon.

70. Zucchini Spaghetti Squash

Ingredients:
- spaghetti squash, seeded and halved lengthwise

- 2 tablespoons olive oil

- 2 small red onion

- 1 zucchini

- ¼ teaspoon salt

- 4 tomatoes, cubed

- ¼ teaspoon ground pepper

- 1 lemon, sliced

Directions:
1. In a baking dish, place the squash halves. Add ¼ cup of water and wrap with a plastic wrap. Put the dish on the microwave and set for 10 minutes on high or until tender. Remove and let it cool.
2. Meanwhile, in a skillet, warm the oil and cook the onion. Sauté for 3 minutes or until translucent. Toss in the zucchini and cook for 5 minutes or until the color turns to brown.
3. Toss in the tomatoes, salt, and pepper. Let it simmer for 10 minutes.

4. Transfer the squash strands into a dish and put the remaining oil. In a pasta bowl, pile the squash in the center and put a dollop of veggie mix around the squash. Add the slices of lemon.

71. Baked Tomatoes with Basil and Tofutti Cheese

Ingredients:
- 3 large tomatoes, cut in half

- ¼ cup fresh herbs (parsley, basil and marjoram)

- ½ cup grated bread crumbs

- ½ cup Tofutti cheese

- 2 cloves garlic, minced

- Pinch of salt

- Pinch of pepper

- 3 tablespoons extra-virgin olive oil

Directions:
1. Preheat the oven to 350 F. Put the tomatoes in a nonstick baking dish.
2. Combine the herbs (parsley, basil, and marjoram), bread crumb, Tofutti cheese, garlic, salt, pepper, and oil in a bowl. Mix well.
3. Sprinkle each of the tomatoes with an equal portion of the mixture. Bake for 30 minutes or until crusty. Serve.

72. Baked Tomatoes with Basil and Tofutti Cheese

Ingredients:
- 3 large tomatoes, cut in half

- ¼ cup fresh herbs (parsley, basil and marjoram)

- ½ cup grated bread crumbs

- ½ cup Tofutti cheese

- 2 cloves garlic, minced

- Pinch of salt

- Pinch of pepper

- 3 tablespoons extra-virgin olive oil

Directions:
1. Preheat the oven to 350 F. Put the tomatoes in a nonstick baking dish.

2. Combine the herbs (parsley, basil, and marjoram), bread crumb, Tofutti cheese, garlic, salt, pepper, and oil in a bowl. Mix well.

3. Sprinkle each of the tomatoes with an equal portion of the mixture. Bake for 30 minutes or until crusty. Serve.

73. Watercress and Arugula Vegan Salad

Ingredients:

Strawberries Preserve
- 5 oz. strawberries, sliced

- 1 tablespoon balsamic vinegar

- 1 ½ tablespoons water

- ½ tablespoon pepper

For the Vinaigrette
- 1 ½ tablespoons white wine vinegar

- 1 ¼ tablespoons lemon juice

- ½ cup extra-virgin olive oil

- 1 ¼ tablespoons black pepper

For the Salad
- 4 oz. watercress leaves

- 4 oz. arugula leaves

- Strawberries, halved

- Pinch black pepper

Directions:

1. To make the strawberry preserves: In a large saucepan, mix the strawberries, vinegar, water, and pepper. Cook at a low for 25 minutes or until the mixture is slightly thickened. When cold, transfer to a bowl and refrigerate.

2. To make the vinaigrette: In a bowl, combine together the vinegar and lemon juice. Whisk the oil and pepper and stir until well combined. Set aside.

3. In a salad bowl, combine the watercress and arugula with the vinaigrette. Dip the cut sides of the strawberry halves in the pepper. Arrange them around the greens. Serve.

74. Nutty Veggie Toast

Ingredients:
- 3 zucchinis, sliced

- 2 leeks, chopped

- 2 tablespoons extra-virgin olive oil

- 2 green peppers, sliced

- Vegan pesto

- 25g vegetarian Parmesan-style cheese, grated

- 50g shelled pistachios

- 1 thick slice white bread

- 1 tablespoon olive oil

Directions:
1. Preheat the oven to 400 F. In a big bowl, combine the zucchini, leeks, and pepper in the oil and pesto.
2. Spread the vegetables in an ovenproof dish and bake for 20 minutes. Stir the veggies and bake for another 20 minutes.
3. In a food processor, mix the Parmesan-style cheese, pistachios, bread, and oil until it becomes a rough crumb. Top the vegetables with the crumbs and bake for another 15 minutes or until crisp and golden brown.

75. Blue Cheese Ice Cream and Red Onion Marmalade

Ingredients:
- 300 ml coconut whipping cream
- 300ml almond milk
- 1 bay leaf
- 2 cloves garlic
- 4 peppercorns
- 1 cup applesauce
- 125g vegetarian soft blue cheese
- 2 tablespoons vegetarian sweet white wine

For the marmalade:
- 1 tablespoon olive oil
- 2 red onions, thinly sliced
- 2 tablespoons sugar
- 1 tablespoon sherry vinegar

Directions:
1. Warm the cream and almond milk together with the garlic and peppercorns. Infuse for 10 minutes. Meanwhile, stir in the applesauce and mix well.

2. Return the mixture to the pan and stir over low heat until it thickens. Add the cheese in batches and pour in the wine. Leave to cool.

3. Put the mixture in a sealable container and freeze. Once partially frozen, beat the mixture and return to the freezer. Repeat this procedure for three times.

4. For the red onion marmalade: In a skillet, fry the onion for 2 minutes until soft. Add the sugar and vinegar until the sugar dissolves. Let it boil for 10 minutes. Store in a jar. You may choose to use it hot or cold.

76. Spinach Loaf

Ingredients:
- 250g almond flour

- 1 ½ teaspoon gluten-free baking powder

- ¼ teaspoon salt

- ¼ teaspoon baking soda

- 2 bunches English spinach, leaves blanched and drained

- 1 cup applesauce

- 60ml coconut milk

- 1 teaspoon lemon juice

- 1 tablespoon olive oil

- 1 tablespoon apple cider vinegar

Directions:
1. Preheat the oven to 345 F and line a loaf tin with baking paper.
2. In a large bowl, combine the almond flour, baking powder, salt, and baking soda. In a food processor, whizz the spinach leaves and toss to the bowl. Combine the applesauce, lemon juice, oil, and apple cider vinegar. Mix thoroughly.

3. Spoon the mixture into the loaf tin and bake on the middle of the rack for 45 minutes. Remove and cool.

77. Cranberry Soup

Ingredients:
- 4 garlic cloves, chopped

- 5 cups vegetable stock

- 5 beets, coarsely chopped, set aside leaves

- Pinch of sea salt

- Pinch of peppercorns

- 2 tablespoons coconut sugar

- 1 cup cranberries

- 1 orange juice, freshly squeezed

- 1 orange zest

- ½ cup fresh dill fronds, chopped

Directions:
5. In a large saucepan, combine garlic, stock, beets, salt, and pepper. Cover the lid and cook on low for 6 hours.

6. Stir in coconut sugar, cranberries, orange juice and zest, and beet leaves. Cover again and cook on high for 30 minutes.

7. Puree the soup in a blender. Transfer to a large soup bow and chill overnight

8. When ready to sue, ladle into individual bowls. Garnish with dill.

Conclusion

Thank you again for reading this book!
I hope this book was able to give you a clearer understanding on how our hunter-gatherer ancestors ate during their time. Although it would be hard to completely imitate their way of consuming healthy produce, it is never too late to start your Paleo journey. Taking on the Paleo route will be all worth it once you have seen improvement in your overall health and the way you see food. You will go for healthier versions instead of settling for convenient fast food.

The next step is to study and follow what you have learned from this book and share the Paleo recipes, tips, and advice with the people you know and care about. Living a healthy lifestyle should not stop at educating yourself on the right foods to eat, it should be shared with those who are still living an unhealthy lifestyle. If you care for a person, spend time sharing this information and watch how their life transforms through you and through the Paleo way of living.

Finally, if you enjoyed this book, then I'd like to ask you for a favor, would you be kind enough to leave a review for this book on Amazon? It'd be greatly appreciated!

www.ingramcontent.com/pod-product-compliance
Lightning Source LLC
Chambersburg PA
CBHW071207280526
45787CB00002B/595